I0839196

HOW TO LOSE WEIGHT FAST AND HEALTHY!

TRICKS AND TIPS TO IMPROVE DIET

CONTENTS

INTRODUCTION 7

HOW TO LOSE 10KG FAST 8

FAST AND EFFICIENT DIETS 18

DIET FOR PEOPLE WITH DIABETES 56

CELEBRITY DIETS 77

TIPS AND RECOMMENDATIONS 90

A TRUE STORY ABOUT THE HARSH REALITY 96
OF EXTRA POUNDS

1

INTRODUCTION

Slimming belts are a growing concern of people regardless of age, gender or origin. Health comes first, and people have come to understand that a healthy person is a person with a normal weight. Achieving and maintaining a healthy weight depends on the foods we eat and the amount of food we eat.

Another important element in achieving and maintaining a healthy weight is exercising. Sport is part of a healthy lifestyle and should be practiced regularly. All people need to be physically active, to exercise regularly because it pretends to the heart and the whole body.

The diet is like a cocktail based on two important ingredients, a healthy diet combined with exercises.

The secret of any diet is to have a lot of will and not give up. In each of us there is an animal, every day there is a strong fight between you and the animal in you, it shows that you are stronger and you defeat the animal in you.

2

HOW TO LOSE 10KG FAST

(1Kg per day)

A fast diet is a diet that manages to burn a large amount of fat in a relatively short period of time. For this you need proper food and self-control. If on day 5 you can't refrain from an ice cream or let yourself be conquered by a lava cake, you can cancel all the effort until then. Determination is the most important word in this period.

Start by cleaning the fridge

Today is the day you say goodbye to Rafael candies. Throw away everything you think causes your appetite or that might tempt you to deviate from your daily plan.

Respect a healthy sleep program

It is proven that sleep is one of the most important factors when it comes to the well-being of our body. Lack of sleep leads to high levels of stress and it is known that stress makes you fat. The chemical parts in our body are disturbed if sleep hormones go crazy. During this diet it is recommended not to have white nights and to sleep 7-8 hours. Preferably go to bed no later than 11 p.m.

Alcohol is not allowed in the fast diet

Avoid going out for 10 days. Social pressure and temptations will help you make mistakes. Alcohol has no nutrient intake, it only adds carbohydrates and a calorie supplement.

You do not have to consume carbohydrates if you want to lose 1 kg per day. Almost any food contains a greater or lesser amount of carbohydrates. It is important to avoid foods such as pasta, bread in large quantities, potatoes, etc. They greatly increase carbohydrate intake and disrupt blood sugar. And if insulin secretion is not enough, the extra sugar reaches the bloodstream.

Eat protein normally

Protein is very important and should not be avoided. In addition to the feeling of satiety offered by them, they also provide essential nutrients to the brain and the whole body.

Try not to eat fat at all

Avoid everything that is greasy as much as possible.

No juices

Juices also contain a lot of sugar. A large number of carbohydrates makes it difficult to establish meals that are somewhat balanced and within the allowed calorie limit.

Fast food or frozen food is forbidden

Street food, pizza and more are strictly forbidden. Their high number of calories and lack of nutrients make any diet impossible. Frozen food loses some of its nutrients and therefore it is good to eat it as fresh as possible.

No fried meat

Any fried food almost doubles its caloric intake. Cook meat only by boiling, steaming or baking (without oil). If you have a tray that has a grill, you can fill the bottom of the tray with water to avoid drying the meat. For a simple tray, you can insert a cup or a heat-resistant bowl filled with water and placed next to or under the oven tray.

No sweets

This should be the first rule in any diet. Sweets contain a large amount of refined sugar.

Drink lots and lots of plain water and teas

No juices or sour drinks. You need to drink as much water as possible. You can't lose weight without consuming a lot of fluids. Water or tea should accompany you both at meals and between meals. If you use a normal glass, it is enough if you drink 15 glasses. It is very important to stay hydrated because water helps the body to function properly and plays an important role in weight loss. During this period it is important to drink more water than usual.

Useful tips in a fast diet

First of all, do not follow any diet if you have not consulted a doctor first. Your health may not allow you such drastic diets. If you feel hungry, drink more water. You can also take calcium, magnesium and multivitamins to strengthen the body. Due to low carbohydrate intake, your condition will suffer. Besides feeling hungry, you will feel slightly depressed and lacking in mood. Multivitamins help a lot on this side.

Menu for ten days to get rid of 10 kg

Before starting the first day, take a picture and stick it in the bathroom on the mirror, on the refrigerator and on the closet in the room. It will help you stay motivated and show you what you are fighting for.

Day 1

Breakfast: 1 cup of coffee (no sugar).

Lunch

- 2 boiled eggs

- 400 g spinach

- 1 tomato

Dinner

- 200g beef

- 1 fresh lettuce

- dressing from a teaspoon of olive oil and the juice of half a lemon

Day 2

Breakfast: 1 cup of coffee (no sugar)

Lunch

- 250 g of ham

- 1 natural yogurt

Dinner

- 200g beef

- 1 fresh lettuce

- dressing from a teaspoon of olive oil and the juice of half a lemon

Day 3

Breakfast: 1 cup of coffee (no sugar) and 1 slice of toast

Lunch

- 2 boiled eggs

- 1 slice of ham

- 1 fresh salad with lemon juice

Dinner

- boiled celery

- 1 tomato

- 1 fresh fruit (apple, pear or orange)

Day 4

Breakfast: 1 cup of coffee (no sugar) and 1 slice of toast

Lunch

- 200 ml of orange juice

- 1 natural yogurt

Dinner

- 1 or proud

- 1 carrot

- 250 g of cottage cheese

Day 5

Breakfast: 1 large carrot

Lunch

- 200 g of boiled cod with lemon juice and 1 teaspoon of butter

Dinner

- 200g beef

- 1 cut celery

Day 6

Breakfast: 1 cup of coffee (no sugar) and 1 slice of toast

Lunch

- 2 boiled eggs

- 1 large carrot

Dinner

- 200g of grilled chicken breast

- 1 fresh lettuce

- dressing from a teaspoon of olive oil and the juice of half a lemon

Day 7

Breakfast: 1 cup of tea (no sugar)

Lunch

- nothing (drink 3l of water, it will help!)

Dinner

- 200 g of honey cutlet

- 1 mar

Day 8

Breakfast: 1 cup of coffee (no sugar)

Lunch

- 2 boiled eggs

- 400 g spinach

- 1 tomato

Dinner

- 200g beef

- 1 salad with oil and lemon juice

Day 9

Breakfast: 1 cup of coffee (no sugar)

Lunch

- 250 g of ham

- 1 natural yogurt

Dinner

- 250 g of grilled beef

- 1 salad with oil and lemon juice

Day 10

Breakfast: 1 cup of coffee (no sugar) and 1 slice of toast

Lunch

- 2 boiled eggs

- 1 slice of ham

- 1 fresh lettuce

- dressing from a teaspoon of olive oil and the juice of half a lemon

Dinner

- 1 boiled celery

- 1 tomato

- 1 fresh fruit (apple, pear or orange)

On day 11, take a picture after the 10 days of treatment and admire the results. Stick this picture next to the others already pasted in the bathroom, on the closet and on the kitchen refrigerator. Every time you want to step crookedly, you will think twice from now on.

It is not the easiest diet to keep, but it is certainly among the fastest.

3

FAST AND EFFICIENT DIETS

1. The Japanese diet

The Japanese diet is based on the consumption of fruits, vegetables, rice and fish. It is a fairly affordable and very promising diet because you lose three kg in three days and if you continue it you can lose ten kg in ten days. A very important aspect of this diet is that it focuses on small portions of food. From what Japanese women and men look like, it is clear that nutrition is what helps them maintain their enviable figure. The daily diet of the Japanese consists of rice, fish, vegetables and fruits served slowly and in small portions.

What you are allowed to eat during the Japanese diet.

Rice, you will need to eat large amounts of rice at almost any meal, including breakfast. The rice must be prepared without butter or oil. It is low in calories and contains complex carbohydrates that provide the feeling of satiety for the last time.

Vegetables, hot peppers, bell peppers, onions, lettuce, tomatoes, radishes, spinach, carrots, mushrooms, beets and many other existing vegetables. They can be prepared in various ways, but for the diet they must be cooked in sauce or steamed to maintain their nutritional qualities. And after finishing the diet they should be included in the daily diet as much as possible.

Fish, it is recommended to eat as many fish as possible: tuna, salmon, mackerel, sardines or herring. Fish rich in Omega 3 fatty acids are preferred because they maintain heart health and improve blood circulation and provide a state of well-being.

Dessert is allowed only on the basis of fruit salad, depending on the season the salad contains assorted fruits.

During this period, some rules must be observed, such as giving up or minimizing alcohol consumption, consuming at least 1.5 liters of water daily and 2 cups of unsweetened green tea.

The main foods are rice, fish and vegetables, and seven different fruits will be eaten during the day. At every meal there should be a food rich in calcium and one containing Omega 3.

3-day diet plan:

Day 1

The first day is the day dedicated to rice. Boil about 250 grams of rice in unsalted water, and after cooling add the fresh juice of half a lemon or an apple put on a grater. The rice prepared in this way is divided into small portions, four or five, which will be consumed throughout the day.

Day 2

The second day is the day dedicated to the consumption of fish. On this day you should eat about 500 grams of fish, salmon, mackerel, tuna, sardines or herring, boiled or grilled. The fish is divided into smaller portions, approximately equal, and will be consumed throughout the day.

Day 3

On the third day you will consume all boiled rice, as on the first day, and if you want you can prepare it mixed with vegetables, of course, also without salt.

If you want to continue the diet, start again in the same order.

Willpower is very important and no matter how difficult it may seem to you, you have to think that achieving the goal of losing weight also requires certain sacrifices. Be a determined person and follow your dream of losing weight and having a perfect figure.

2. Yogurt diet

The yogurt diet is a diet that is based on the consumption of yogurt, it is a cheap diet and quite easy to follow. This diet is an emergency solution for cases when you want to lose weight quickly before an important event, a social event or a wedding. Yogurt can be successfully integrated into the daily diet because it has multiple health and silhouette benefits. This diet is based on lactic acid bacteria from fermented dairy products and the beneficial effects they have on the intestinal flora, facilitates the rapid digestion of food and the efficient elimination of toxins. Another reason why yogurt is good for weight loss is the high calcium intake that stimulates the appetite. The amino acids in yogurt help burn fat. This diet is recommended to be followed for a period of three days and during this time in addition to yogurt can be eaten fresh fruit and low-fat meat. Avoid eating sugary yogurts such as fruit yogurts. You can make such yogurts at home from yogurt and pieces of fresh fruit without other ingredients.

Diet plan for three days

Day 1

For breakfast, serve a plain yogurt, in which you add fruits such as raspberries, blueberries, apple pieces or a plain low-fat yogurt, along with a portion of whole grains, such as oatmeal.

For lunch, opt for vegetables cooked with a little olive oil and rice. Do not use spices other than salt and pepper. The dessert can consist of a yogurt in which to add a few pieces of fruit.

For dinner, eat a salad with boiled chicken or simply cooked in the oven with grated carrots, mixed with low-fat yogurt.

Day 2

For breakfast, eat a cucumber salad with yogurt.

For lunch, opt for turkey meat cooked in a little olive oil in the oven or on the grill, and for the garnish choose a portion of au gratin mushrooms, tomatoes and bell peppers, all mixed with yogurt.

For dinner, combine a portion of berries with a small yogurt.

Day 3

For breakfast, combine a portion of cheese under 5% fat, along with a few pieces of apple, cinnamon and a few teaspoons of yogurt.

Lunch can consist of a portion of fish fillets, lettuce or leurd, iceberg lettuce, arugula with green onions and radishes, yogurt and cucumber (you can add, for more taste and a little mustard).

For dinner, opt for 100 grams of cooked pasta, possibly rice noodles, combined with a teaspoon of olive oil, a bell pepper cut into pieces, a boiled egg and a yogurt.

It is recommended that yogurt, either in the form of sana, kefir or skim yogurt, be present in the 3 main meals, in different forms. Also, if you have trouble sleeping, bowel problems, or acute weakness during the treatment, it is advisable to stop the diet immediately. It is advisable to respect the consumption of at least 2 liters of water per day, and the consumption of green tea (one cup per day) can help speed up the metabolism. Also, regular exercise, of moderate intensity, at least 30 minutes a day, can increase the beneficial effects of the yogurt diet.

3. Mayo Diet

The Mayo diet is an easy way to lose weight, but also an effective way to improve your lifestyle. In addition to a healthy menu, the Mayo Clinic diet promises to help you lose 5 pounds in just 13 days. And because it involves eating vegetables, fruits, grains and lean meats, it's also a cheap way to stay healthy and fit. This diet is built in the form of a Mayo food pyramid, which helps you focus on healthy foods and helps you lose weight.

The food pyramid of the diet is based on fruits and vegetables, then carbohydrates, proteins / dairy products, fats and last floor, sweets. If the portions in the groups at the base of the pyramid can be generous, the further we go towards the top, the smaller the portions become. Free fruits and vegetables, whole grains, vegetable and dairy proteins and healthy fats can be eaten.

Fast Mayo diet for days

Day 1

Breakfast: a coffee with a maximum of one sugar cube.

Lunch: 400 grams of spinach (boiled), 2 boiled eggs and a tomato.

Dinner: 200 grams of beef steak with a salad (with oil and lemon juice).

Day 2

Breakfast: identical the first day.

Lunch: 250 grams of ham and a box of natural yogurt.

Dinner: 200 grams of beef steak and a salad (with oil and lemon juice).

Day 3

Breakfast: a cup of coffee with a sugar cube and a slice of toast.

Lunch: 2 boiled eggs (countries), a slice of ham and a salad.

Dinner: a tomato, a boiled celery and a fresh fruit (apple, orange or pear).

Day 4

Breakfast: identical to day 3.

Lunch: a box of natural yogurt and 200 ml of orange juice.

Dinner: a boiled egg (hard), 250 grams of cottage cheese and a carrot.

Day 5

Breakfast: a large grated carrot.

Lunch: 250 grams of cod (boiled) with lemon juice and a teaspoon of butter.

Dinner: 200 grams of beef steak and a grated celery.

Day 6

Breakfast: identical to day 3.

Lunch: 2 boiled eggs and a large carrot.

Dinner: half a chicken and a salad with oil and lemon juice.

Day 7

Breakfast: a cup of sugar-free tea.

Lunch: just plenty of plain water.

Dinner: 200 grams of lamb chop and an apple.

Then, on days 8-13, the menu on days 1-6 is repeated. It is important to drink as much plain water between meals daily (on average 2-3 liters), to avoid alcoholic beverages and to follow the diet without deviations. If for more than 6 days you fail to strictly follow the diet of this diet, then you need to stop it and resume it.

4. Diet with apples

The apple diet is an easy diet to follow. This diet helps you get an enviable figure and has many beneficial effects on the whole body. It involves eating as many apples as possible in a day, along with a little low-fat cheese, lean meat and water. Cheap and beneficial in terms of health. The apple diet promises to get rid of not only weight, but also toxins. Apples are the most suitable fruits in diets because they have few calories, an average apple has around 80 calories, are rich in vitamins and minerals, contain a lot of fiber, help digestion, lower cholesterol, are full, cut the appetite food and removes toxins from the body.

Apple diet - menu for 5 days

Day 1: breakfast, lunch, dinner - apples (not more than 1.5 kilograms)

Day 2: breakfast - 2 apples, lunch - an apple and a vegetable salad with two slices of low-fat cheese, sprinkled only with lemon juice, dinner - 3 apples

Day 3: breakfast - an apple, a slice of wholemeal bread and a slice of lean turkey ham, lunch - an apple, a salad made only from half lettuce, 2 grated carrots and half an onion, dinner - 3 apples .

Day 4: breakfast - an apple, a slice of lean chicken or turkey ham and a slice of wholemeal bread, lunch - an apple, a salad of boiled vegetables (excluding potatoes) with 200 gr canned tuna, dinner - 3 apples and a bowl of low-fat milk and whole grains.

Day 5: breakfast - an apple, a boiled egg and a slice of wholemeal bread, lunch - an apple and a salad of vegetables with 200 g of beef or chicken without skin, dinner - 3 apples.

5. Country diet

The Country diet is perfect for those people who want to lose 4-5 kilograms, without starving. Many people resort to this diet when they want to lose extra pounds, no wonder this diet is a success.

This diet can be the perfect weight loss regimen, especially when you want to have energy. Thus, you will be able to enjoy a beautiful and active life in the future. Diets that have a lot of restrictions tend to make us tired, it is not very pleasant to stay without food for days, just to look good. Maybe the first days will be a little more difficult, because you will only eat fruits and vegetables, but you can eat as you please, that is, every time you are hungry. Of course you don't have to exaggerate. The next day of the Country diet, you will become familiar with eating raw and steamed vegetables, but it would be advisable to avoid beans. There is good news, you can consume: lentils, chickpeas, broccoli, carrots, raw goulash, etc. So don't say you have nothing to eat.

Country diet - menu by days:

Day 1

You will only eat fruit, you can eat it whenever you are hungry

Day 2

Raw and steamed vegetables, every time you're hungry

Day 3

You are also allowed fruits and vegetables, as you like.

Day 4

Bananas and milk, ie around 5-6 bananas and 5-6 glasses of milk (the vegetable one is even better).

Day 5

About 300 grams of baked beef, tomato salad

Day 6

About 300 grams of beef and stewed vegetables

Day 7

Brown rice with vegetables and fruit juices, 2 times a day (ie at lunch and dinner, in the morning you will eat fruit salad and cereals)

The Country diet does not require a significant effort, but after this period you will lose about 5 kilograms. Don't forget to drink plenty of water and do sports. The first few days may be harder, but you can be sure it's well worth the effort. Enjoy your diet and trust yourself, do not overdo it and you will see results quickly.

6. Crono Diet

The Crono diet is also called the clockwise diet, it is a metabolic chrono diet that guarantees the loss of 5-7 kilograms in two weeks respecting the principles of a balanced and healthy diet without causing hunger. The most important thing is when we eat. This idea is the basis of the diet created by Alain Debalos in 1986. After 30 years, the diet that recommends eating food at the same hours every day has returned to the present.

You lose 5-7 kilograms in two weeks and this without giving up your favorite foods, you eat everything your heart desires and you manage not to gain weight, but also to lose the extra kilograms. All you have to do is be as organized as possible and follow the same meal schedule every day. Specifically, follow the Crono diet and you will lose weight almost miraculously.

Each of us has an inner clock that works 24 hours a day. It helps the body get used to climate change, sleep and even eating. In other words, not only what we assimilate through food is essential, but also when we assimilate the food we eat. More specifically, mealtimes influence the regulation of metabolism and weight gain, the way we fight diseases caused by obesity and, as well, can have an impact on our sleep cycle.

We must follow the same diet. It sounds complicated, but it's not at all. The researchers analyzed the subject at length and, following the studies made, drew some conclusions about the hours at which it is optimal to eat. Thus, it was concluded that people who take lunch late, after 3 pm, lose less weight than those who eat breakfast earlier. In addition, when we eat only between 6 and 19, we assimilate fewer calories (244 less) than if we continued to eat in the evening. This is possible because there are fewer hours in which we eat and thus assimilate fewer calories, but also because the moment we eat decides the weight we have.

A longer overnight fast (we do not eat late in the evening) helps to lose body fat because the body has enough time to reach the state of ketosis, which indicates that the body begins to use fat to gain energy, so we lose weight.

Regarding breakfast, a study claims that people who eat breakfast have a lower amount of body fat and a lower appetite to eat snacks than those who do not eat in the morning. Another study found that obese women who eat more in the first part of the day than in the last have lost more weight and have a more alert metabolism. However, if we assimilate a higher number of calories in the morning, it is not mandatory to consume a lower number of calories in the rest of the day.

Regular meals are good for your figure. When we eat at fixed hours, this sets the body for a certain schedule. Changing meal times causes the body to adjust, but this adjustment takes several days. Regular meals also play a key role in long-term body weight. Usually, the body requires food once every three or five hours, this interval being optimal to provide the body with the daily needs, not starving it.

When we consider a diet, we immediately think about the quality of the food. But the time we eat is as important as everything we eat. If we turn our internal clock upside down due to lack of sleep, for example, we end up eating at inappropriate hours and, implicitly, gaining weight. Insomniacs tend to eat more fast food, sour juices, fatty foods and less fruits and vegetables. If two people eat the same number of calories, but at different times, the one who consumed them after 8 pm gained more weight than the other.

The best food program is the one that suits your lifestyle. But the chrono diet recommends following a few common sense rules that work wonders for your figure.

Regular crono diet

Eat at the same hours every day.

Eat breakfast over other meals during the day.

Lunch should not be served late, and dinner should not be too substantial.

Refrain from eating at night or after 7 p.m.

Respect the hours of sleep and do not sleep with the light on. Exposure to light upsets your internal clock, which makes you put the yam in the fridge at midnight.

Eat protein within 45 minutes of exercising to help your body begin the process of rebuilding muscles affected by exertion.

Recommended menu in fixed hours mode

Breakfast

One hour after waking up, but no later than 9 o'clock, consume fat and protein. Recommended foods for the first hours of the day: dairy (milk, cheese, yogurt, butter), protein (eggs, chicken or turkey, ham), slow sugars (wholemeal bread) and liquids (water, tea, even coffee) .

Lunch

At noon, it is good to satisfy your need for sugar, protein and starch. Recommended foods for lunch: meat or fish, pasta, rice, wheat, fruits, vegetables. After 2 pm, avoid desserts and even bread, if you want impressive results.

Dinner

Given that in the evening, ie in the absence of natural light, the body no longer secretes the enzymes necessary for digestion, we give up the meal after dark or we limit ourselves to the consumption of fiber and protein. Recommended foods in the last part of the day: vegetables, fish, seafood.

This diet can be kept for a longer period of time until the desired weight is reached and it is very important that this diet becomes a lifestyle.

7. Dissociated diet 333

This diet is a popular weight loss method because it helps you lose weight in a very short time. The "333" diet means 3 days of meat, 3 days of fruits and vegetables, 3 days of dairy. Under this regime, there is no limit on quantity. The meat must be steamed or grilled.

Permitted foods and forbidden foods in the dissociated diet 333

During the dissociated diet, avoid alcohol, carbonated juices, caffeine and sugar. Because the diet supports proper digestion, snacks are not encouraged and a break of at least four hours between main meals is recommended. During this time, the stomach has enough time to process the food ingested at the previous meal and prepare for the next. Dinner must always be taken before 7 p.m.

Drink at least two liters of water daily and add to your program at least 30 minutes of exercise, in any form. On days when your diet limits you to eating fruits or vegetables, you may feel a slight muscle weakness due to the lack of protein on the menu. In these cases you can opt for easy 40-minute walks.

Avoid drinking water 30 minutes before a meal or during a meal because liquids dilute gastric juices and make digestion difficult.

3 days dedicated to fruits and vegetables, except for carbohydrate-rich foods such as bananas, grapes, dried fruits, candied fruits, potatoes, peas and beans. Vegetables can be steamed, grilled or pan-fried with a little water. The use of oil is excluded.

3 days dedicated to dairy products, it is recommended to consume only skim milk.

3 days dedicated to meat, you are allowed to eat any type of poultry (legs, chest, muscles), lean chicken or turkey ham, seafood, fish and beef. You must remove any traces of fat or skin before eating the meat, which you can boil or steam or grill. You

are also allowed to season with any type of spices and aromatic herbs.

8. Indian diet

The Indian diet is a nutritional plan designed specifically to reduce body fat levels and total weight in just 7 days. This is the best vegetarian diet to lose weight. This vegetarian diet plan for weight loss does not only consist in weight loss itself, it is also a way to keep the body in normal parameters.

The diet encourages the consumption of vegetables and fruits, which will help increase the metabolic rate. Vegetarian diets and weight loss go hand in hand. It is the healthiest and fastest way to lose extra pounds.

The Indian diet is a good way to detoxify the body, avoid eating unhealthy foods such as fats, processed proteins and unhealthy carbohydrates. This is an effective way to get rid of toxins accumulated in the body.

Indian diet: 7 day plan

Day 1

Being the first day, this will always be the hardest, because only fruit will be consumed. All fruits can be eaten, except grapes, bananas, lychees and mangoes, in any quantity. However, higher consumption of watermelon, apples, oranges, pomegranates, strawberries and melons is suggested. It can be eaten 20 times a day, strictly fruit.

Breakfast (8.30 AM) - 1 medium apple, 1 glass of water

Morning snack (10.30) - 1 bowl of melon, 1 glass of water

Lunch (12.00 at noon) - 2 slices of watermelon, 2 glasses of water

Afternoon snack (16:00) - 1 orange, 1 glass of water

Evening snack (6.30) - 1 pear, 1 glass of water

Dinner (20.00) - 1 guava, 1/2 grapefruit, 2 glasses of water

Day 2

The next day is the day of all vegetables. You can eat as many vegetables to satiety, but it is important that they are cooked or raw. You can start the day with a boiled potato and a tablespoon of butter, along with tea. This is done to provide the body with enough energy and carbohydrates for the day.

Breakfast (8.30 AM) - 1 medium boiled potato, melted with 1 teaspoon butter

Morning snack (10.30 AM) - 1 bowl of cabbage and lettuce, 1 glass of water

Lunch (12.00) - 1 cucumber, 1 onion, 1/2 carrot, 2 glasses of water

Afternoon snack (16.00) - 1 cup boiled broccoli, 1/2 cup peppers, 2 glasses of water

Evening snack (6.30 PM) - 1 cup boiled cauliflower, 1 glass of water

Dinner (20.00) - Mix of carrots, beets, broccoli and green beans, 2 glasses of water

Day 3

Day 3 is a combination of days 1 and 2. You can eat the mentioned fruits and vegetables in any quantity and drink a lot of water. Potatoes should be avoided on day 3 as a sufficient amount of carbohydrates is obtained from the fruit. The system is set to burn excess weight. Appetites can try to dominate, but weight loss and the best results must be the goals that no one should deviate from.

Breakfast (8.30 AM) - 1 bowl of melon or 1 apple, 2 glasses of water

Morning snack (10.30 AM) - 1 pear, pineapple slices, 2 glasses of water

Lunch (12.00) - 1 bowl with a mix of cucumber, onion, carrots, lettuce, 2 glasses of water

Afternoon snack (16.00) - 1 orange or 1/2 grapefruit and 1 glass of water

Evening snack (6.30 PM) - 1 pear or 1 guava

Dinner (20.00) - 1 bowl of boiled broccoli, 1/2 boiled beets, 1/2 cup raw papaya, 2 glasses of water

Day 4

On the fourth day of the vegetarian diet for weight loss, you can eat up to 6 bananas for the whole day. You can drink up to 4 glasses of milk. Although bananas can make you fat, in this diet they act as a source of potassium and sodium for the body. Due to low salt consumption, bananas will do their job efficiently.

Breakfast (8.30 AM) - 2 bananas, 1 glass of milk

Morning snack (10.30) - Banana mix with 1 cup of milk

Lunch (12.00) - 1 bowl of vegetable soup made with cabbage, carrots and onions

Afternoon snack (4.00 PM) - Banana shake made with 1 banana and 1 glass of milk

Dinner (20.00) - 2 bananas and 1 glass of milk

Drink 8 to 10 glasses of water during the day.

Day 5

Day 5 is a holiday because you can have a tasty meal. You can eat tomatoes, cabbage, sprouts and cottage cheese. You can also add pieces of soy to the table or prepare a tasty soup with the mentioned ingredients. Water intake should also be increased on day 5.

Breakfast (8.30 AM) - 2 tomatoes, a bowl of boiled red beans seasoned with salt, pepper and lemon, 2 glasses of water

Morning snack (10.30 AM) - a cup of tofu or curd, 2 glasses of water

Lunch (12.00) - a bowl of cheese, 2 tomatoes, spinach, 2 glasses of water

Afternoon snack (4.30 am) - lettuce with onion, lemon juice, pepper and a pinch of salt, 2 glasses of water

Dinner (8.00 PM) - Curry made from soy / vegetable soup, cucumber and tomato salad from 1 cucumber and 2 tomatoes, 2 glasses of water.

Day 6

This day is a little different from day 5. It looks like the day before, except for the tomatoes. Tasty soup and plenty of water should help during the day. Vegetables will provide vitamins and fiber to the body. At this point, changes in the body will be observed.

Breakfast (8.30 AM) - 1 bowl of mixed vegetables, boiled or with sauce, 2 glasses of water

Morning snack (10.30 AM) - medium boiled beans with 1 cube of seasoned tomatoes with a pinch of salt and other spices, 2 glasses of water

Lunch (12.00) - 1 cup boiled brown rice, 1 bowl of vegetable soup, 2 glasses of water

Afternoon snack (4.00 PM) - 1 apple, 1 glass of water

Evening snack (6.30) - 1 small bowl of boiled lentils, seasoned with salt and lemon juice, 1 glass of water

Dinner (20.00) - 1 bowl of mixed boiled vegetables, 1 glass of water

Day 7

Last day of the diet plan. This is the most important day. You can consume fresh fruit juice, a cup of brown rice or other vegetables. Do not forget about water consumption.

Breakfast (8.30 AM) - 1 bowl of melon, 1 glass of water

Morning snack (10.30 AM) - A handful of fresh or frozen fruit or 1 carrot, 1 glass of water

Lunch (12.00) - 1 cup boiled brown rice, 1 bowl of dried vegetables, 2 glasses of water

Afternoon snack (16.00) - 1 apple or 1 pear, 1 glass of water

Evening snack (6.30) - 1 guava, 1 glass of water

Dinner (20.00) - 1 bowl of mixed vegetable soup, 2 glasses of water

It combines the Indian diet with exercise, increasing in intensity throughout the day.

Basic rules. What vegetables can be eaten.

• Potatoes (only for breakfast on day 2) - The starch present in chilled boiled potatoes turns into resistant starch, which promotes the oxidation of fats and reduces abdominal fat.

• Cucumber - This is one of the best low calorie and non-starchy vegetables for weight loss. Half sliced cucumber contains only 10 calories.

• Salad - one of the healthiest vegetables, which is low in calories and rich in vitamins and fiber.

• Cabbage - rich in vitamin C and antioxidants, cabbage helps increase immunity.

• Broccoli - the sulforaphane found in broccoli fights body fats. This low-calorie vegetable is an important source of fiber and calcium

• Bell peppers - The metabolism-stimulating dihydrocapsiate present in bell peppers promotes fat burning.

• Onions - Quercetin, the flavonoid found in onions activates proteins in the body, burns stored fat and prevents the formation of new fat cells.

• Spinach - This leafy green vegetable is loaded with proteins that promote lean muscle mass and promote calorie burning.

• Carrots - Carrots are loaded with beta-carotene and fiber.

• Cauliflower - This cruciferous vegetable is loaded with fiber, folic acid and vitamin C.

9. Keto Diet

The Keto or ketogenic diet is based on a diet rich in fats and proteins and with very few carbohydrates. By majorly reducing the body's intake of carbohydrates and replacing them with fats, the body is introduced into a metabolic state called ketosis. When the body is in the state of ketosis, fats become the main supplier of energy to the body, which is pleasing to most cells in the body. When we eat less than 50 grams of carbohydrates a day, the body enters the state of ketosis, a state that offers multiple benefits to the body, such as: reducing the level of sugar and insulin in the blood and reducing body fat. The ketogenic diet may be perfect for overweight, diabetic people or those looking to improve their metabolic health, but more unsuitable for performance athletes or those who want to develop muscle or gain weight.

Foods to be reduced or eliminated in the ketogenic diet:

Sugar: Juices, fruit juices, purees, cakes, ice cream, candy and sweets

Starchy cereals: products based on wheat, rice, pasta and cereals

Fruit: all fruits except small portions of berries

Beans or vegetables grains: peas, beans, lentils, chickpeas

Vegetables and roots: potatoes, sweet potatoes, carrots, parsley

Low fat or dietary products are highly processed and often high in carbohydrates.

Some spices or sauces often contain sugar and unhealthy fats

Unhealthy fats: limit the intake of processed vegetable oils

Alcohol: Due to its carbohydrate content, many alcoholic beverages can get you out of your ketosis state.

You should base most meals around these foods:

Meat: red meat, steak, ham, sausages, bacon, chicken and turkey.

Fatty fish: such as salmon, trout, tuna and mackerel.

Eggs

Butter

Cheese: Raw cheese (cedar, goat, sour cream, cheese with mold or mozzarella).

Walnuts and seeds: almonds, walnuts, flax seeds, pumpkin seeds, chia seeds

Healthy oils: Extra virgin olive oil, coconut oil and avocado oil.

Avocado: Whole avocado or fresh guacamole.

Low carb vegetables: most green, red, onion, pepper vegetables

Spices: You can use salt, pepper and various herbs and healthy spices.

Always try to vary vegetables and meat in the long run, because each type offers different nutrients and health benefits.

BENEFITS

The keto diet is recommended when we want to lose weight and tone up, with the great advantage that you will not feel hungry, unlike other diets for weight loss.

People who used a keto diet lost 2.2 times more weight than those who used a low-fat, low-calorie diet, and their triglyceride and cholesterol levels also improved.

Example menu for a week

MONTHS

breakfast: bacon + eggs + spinach

lunch: grilled chicken + salad (leaves) + feta cheese

dinner: salmon + asparagus cooked with butter

TUESDAY

breakfast: egg omelette + tomatoes + goat cheese / sheep / cow + basil

lunch: almond milk milkshake + peanut butter + cocoa powder

dinner: meatballs + cheddar cheese + vegetables

WEDNESDAY

breakfast: ketogenic milshake: almond milk + peanut butter + cocoa powder

lunch: shrimp salad with olive oil and avocado

dinner: pork with parmesan + broccoli + salad (leaves)

THURSDAY

breakfast: avocado omelette + hot peppers + onions + spices

lunch: a handful of nuts + asparagus + avocado + spices

dinner: chicken stuffed with cheese + vegetable salad

FRIDAY

breakfast: fat-free yogurt without sugar + peanut butter + cocoa lunch: beef cooked in coconut oil + vegetables with low glycemic index

dinner: bacon + eggs + cheese

SATURDAY

breakfast: omelet + cheese + vegetables

lunch: slices of ham + slices of cheese + nuts

dinner: fish + eggs + spinach, cooked in coconut oil

SUNDAY

breakfast: fried eggs + bacon + mushrooms

lunch: meat + cheese + avocado + vegetables

dinner: steak chicken + eggs + salad (leaves)

Keto diet - snack allowed

a handful of nuts, almonds, pistachios, macadamia nuts

pumpkin or sunflower seeds

olive cheese

a boiled egg

2 dark chocolate cubes

milkshake with almond milk

berries

10. The Mediterranean diet

Many people love the lifestyle of the people of the Mediterranean area. It is impossible not to like the way they are, especially since the peoples on the shores of the Mediterranean generally have a high life expectancy compared to the rest of Europe. One of the secrets of such a lasting life is nutrition. Mediterranean countries have a high life expectancy due to a diet based on vegetables and fish and a lack of unhealthy fats.

Many doctors and nutritionists recommend the Mediterranean diet for its ability to prevent disease and keep people healthy for longer. The Mediterranean diet places great emphasis on vegetables, fruits and whole grains. In addition, it does not contain as much dairy and meat as Western foods.

Basically, those who want to adopt such a diet must consume what is usually eaten by people in the Mediterranean region. In short, a traditional Mediterranean diet contains a generous portion of fresh produce, whole grains and legumes, as well as some fats and fish meat.

The Mediterranean diet consists of foods that people traditionally ate in countries such as Italy and Greece in the 1960s. Research has shown that these people were exceptionally healthy compared to Americans, for example. In addition, due to their diet, these people had a low risk of developing more lifestyle diseases.

The benefits of the Mediterranean diet

Nutrition influences many aspects of health, including brain health. Therefore, a healthy diet can improve the ability to think, store and process information as we age. Specialists have shown that the Mediterranean diet stimulates brain health and improves heart health.

According to several recent researches, the Mediterranean diet can support the weight loss process and can help prevent strokes, heart attacks, type 2 diabetes and premature death.

There is no precise way you can follow the Mediterranean diet, because there are several countries in this area, and the diets may be different depending on the state. One thing is for sure, however, the Mediterranean diet is mainly based on:

- dairy and fish in moderate quantities

- a wide variety of vegetables, fruits and whole grains

- Healthy fats such as nuts, seeds and olive oil

- very little white meat and red meat

- A few eggs

- red wine in moderation

Foods recommended in the Mediterranean diet

It is recommended to eat fish and seafood at least twice a week. The Mediterranean lifestyle does not just mean a healthy diet. It also involves regular physical activity, sharing meals with loved ones, and enjoying life. You should definitely rely on these healthy, unprocessed Mediterranean foods:

- Vegetables: cabbage, spinach, tomatoes, broccoli, onions, Brussels sprouts, cauliflower, carrots, cucumbers, etc.

- Fruits: bananas, apples, oranges, strawberries, pears, grapes, melons, dates, figs, peaches, etc.

- Walnuts and seeds: walnuts, almonds, macadamia nuts, cashews, hazelnuts, sunflower seeds, pumpkin seeds, etc.

- Tubers: potatoes, turnips, yams, sweet potatoes, etc.

- Legumes: peas, beans, lentils, peanuts, legumes, chickpeas, etc.

- Whole grains: brown rice, whole oats, rye, whole wheat, corn, barley, buckwheat, whole wheat bread and pasta.

- Fish and seafood: sardines, salmon, trout, mackerel, tuna, shrimp, crab, oysters, mussels, mussels, etc.

- Herbs and spices: basil, mint, garlic, rosemary, cinnamon, sage, nutmeg, pepper, etc.

- Healthy fats: extra virgin olive oil, olives, avocado and avocado oil.

Whole foods, consisting of a single ingredient, are the key to good health.

What can you drink if you choose the Mediterranean diet

Obviously, water is the favorite drink in the Mediterranean diet. However, it is well-known that Mediterranean people usually consume about a glass of red wine a day. However, this is completely optional, and wine should be avoided by people who have problems with alcohol consumption. In addition, coffee and tea are completely allowed. However, sugary drinks and fruit juices, which have a high sugar content, should be avoided.

Foods to eat in moderation in the Mediterranean diet

In addition to those listed above, you can include the following foods in your diet, although they should be eaten in moderation:

- Poultry: chicken, duck, turkey, etc.

- Dairy products: yogurt, cheese, yogurt, etc.

- Eggs: chicken eggs, duck and quail.

-Pork is also allowed, but in small quantities and extremely rarely.

Foods to avoid in the Mediterranean diet

The chapter on foods banned in any form in the Mediterranean diet includes these unhealthy foods and ingredients:

- Refined wheat products: white bread, pasta made with refined wheat, etc.

- Refined oils: canola oil, soybean oil, cottonseed oil and others.

- Added sugar: juices, ice cream, candy, sugar and much more.

- Trans fats: these are found in margarine and various processed foods.

- Processed meat: processed sausages, hot dogs, etc.

- Highly processed foods: Any product whose label states "low fat" or "dietary" or that appears to be made in a factory.

Nutritionists also recommend that you read food labels carefully if you want to completely avoid these unhealthy ingredients.

Healthy Mediterranean snacks

First of all, it is essential to know that you should not eat more than 3 meals a day. But if you get hungry between meals, you have a lot of healthy snacks:

- a handful of nuts

- a fruit

- carrots or baby carrots

- some berries or grapes

- yogurt

- apple slices with almond butter.

How to choose Mediterranean food when going to a restaurant

If you do not have the time or desire to cook, it is very simple to compose a Mediterranean style meal at the restaurant.

- Choose fish or seafood as the main dish.

- Ask the cooks to prepare your food in extra virgin olive oil.

- Consume only wholemeal bread, with olive oil instead of butter.

How to organize a simple shopping list

Most of the time, it is a good idea to shop at nearby stores. Usually, whole foods can be found in these stores. Always try to buy the least processed products. Organic foods are the best, provided you can afford them without much effort.

The ideal list of products to add to your shopping cart includes:

- Vegetables: carrots, onions, broccoli, spinach, cabbage, garlic, etc.

- Fruits: apples, bananas, oranges, grapes, etc.

- Berries: blueberries, strawberries, etc.

- Wheat: wholemeal bread, wholemeal pasta, etc.

- Frozen vegetables: choose mixtures with healthy vegetables.

- Legumes: lentils, beans, etc.

- yogurt.

- Walnuts: walnuts, almonds, cashews, etc.

- Seeds: pumpkin seeds, sunflower seeds, etc.

- Spices: sea salt, pepper, cinnamon, turmeric, etc.

- Cheese.

- Fish: salmon, mackerel, sardines, trout.

- Shrimp and shellfish.

- Potatoes and sweet potatoes.

- Chicken.

- Eggs.

- Olives.

- Extra virgin olive oil.

It is also recommended to remove from the list all unhealthy temptations, such as soft drinks, candy, ice cream, white bread, pastries, biscuits and processed foods. If you only have healthy food at home, you will eat healthy food.

Example menu for a week. You can adjust portions and food options according to the needs of your body and according to your preferences.

Months:

Breakfast: yogurt with strawberries and oatmeal.

Lunch: focaccia with olives or pita with lots of vegetable salad (salad leaves, cucumbers, peppers, cherry tomatoes sprinkled with oil and lemon) with grilled squid.

Dinner: A large tuna salad with a hard boiled egg, sweet corn or lentils, arugula leaves, iceberg, lettuce, tomatoes, onions, green garlic, with olive and lemon oil dressing, spices

Tuesday:

Breakfast: oatmeal (ie breakfast cereals, soaked) with raisins.

Lunch: Tuna salad (for example, what you have left from the previous evening).

Dinner: Salad with tomatoes, olives and feta cheese, sprinkled with olive oil, pepper and coriander.

Wednesday:

Breakfast: omelette with vegetables, tomatoes and onions. Only one fruit is recommended.

Lunch: a large salad with several kinds of leaves, tomatoes, onions, sliced pumpkin pieces, with cheese and fresh vegetables.

Dinner: Mediterranean lasagna, ie cooked without meat, only with chopped vegetables, to which you can add diced mushrooms, possibly the composition drawn in a pan, with olive oil and seasoned with fresh and dried herbs

Thursday:

Breakfast: yogurt with slices of fruit and a few nuts (cashews, macadamia nuts, Brazilian nuts, peanuts or pumpkin seeds or sunflower).

Lunch: a portion of lasagna (left over from last night's dinner).

Dinner: Baked or grilled salmon, served with brown rice and vegetable garnish.

Friday:

Breakfast: eggs and vegetables, slightly fried in olive oil.

Lunch: yogurt with strawberries, 50g oatmeal and 5 nuts.

Dinner: grilled lamb chops, with lettuce, flavored with chives or green onions, lime dressing and extra virgin olive oil

Saturday:

Breakfast: oat bran porridge with a handful of raisins, nuts and diced apple, cinnamon.

Lunch: seafood - grilled octopus - with pan-fried vegetables (zucchini, thinly sliced sweet potato, eggplant, capsicum) and mozzarella.

Dinner: Mediterranean pizza, made with whole wheat flour, in an extremely thin top, and on top with a little cheese, vegetables, fresh arugula and olives.

Sunday:

Breakfast: omelette with vegetables, cherry tomatoes and olives.

Lunch: two leftover slices from last night's pizza, sprinkled with fresh extra virgin olive oil

Dinner: grilled chicken or turkey, with pan-fried vegetables (zucchini, eggplant, peppers, thin slices of cucumber, small bouquets of broccoli).

4

DIET FOR PEOPLE WITH DIABETES

The role of diet for diabetes

There are several aspects to the treatment of diabetes, and each of them has a very important role. One of these aspects is the diet. In other words, the patient who has been diagnosed with diabetes must follow a special diet that meets his nutritional needs and helps him keep his blood sugar under control, and the patient's diet will work with the medications prescribed by the doctor for diabetes, regular exercise and maintaining a normal body weight.

Glucose level control through diet

When you overeat foods high in calories and fat, your body responds by creating an unwanted increase in blood glucose (sugar) levels. If blood glucose is not kept under control and is not checked (blood glucose measurement is an extremely important aspect), this can lead to serious problems such as hyperglycemia (extremely high and dangerous blood glucose levels) and to long-term complications such as nerve, kidney and heart damage. You can keep your blood glucose level (blood sugar) at a safe value, making healthier food choices and following your eating habits, and where appropriate, making small changes for the better.

Weight control through food

For most patients with diabetes and weight loss can ease the effort, meaning that it will be easier for the patient to keep their blood sugar under control and enjoy other health benefits. If your doctor tells you that you need to lose weight or keep your weight under control, a diabetes diet gives you a well-organized way and a nutrient-rich method to achieve your goal safely.

Nutrition and food preparation in the diet for diabetes

A diet for diabetes is based on the fact that the patient must eat three main meals a day at regular times. This helps the body make better use of the insulin it produces or takes through drug treatment. It is important to improve your eating habits by choosing the right sized portions that suit your needs, depending on your figure and weight, but also depending on your level of physical activity.

Recommended foods for diabetes

The main idea in a diabetes diet is to make those calories you eat really matter by choosing nutritious (nutritious) foods, such as:

• healthy carbohydrates, ie complex ones such as fruits, vegetables, whole grains, legumes and skim dairy products;

• foods rich in dietary fiber, such as vegetables, fruits, nuts, legumes (beans, peas and lentils), whole wheat flour and wheat bran;

• healthy fish, whose flesh protects your heart; Ideally, you should eat fish meat twice a week, such as salmon, mackerel, tuna, sardines and other types of fish rich in Omega-3 fatty acids.

• "good" fats, meaning eating those foods that contain monounsaturated and polyunsaturated fats, which can help lower your cholesterol; these are avocados, almonds, pecans, Romanian walnuts, olives, olive oil, peanut oil and canola oil (rapeseed).

Healthy carbohydrates in the diet for diabetes

Healthy carbohydrates are very important in the diet for diabetes. During digestion, sugars (simple carbohydrates) and starch (complex carbohydrates) break down into blood glucose. You need to focus on healthy carbohydrates, such as fruits, vegetables, whole grains, legumes (beans of different colors, peas and lentils) and low-fat dairy products.

High fiber foods in the diet for diabetes

High fiber foods should be included in the diet for diabetes. Dietary fiber (or dietary fiber) includes all parts of plant foods that your body cannot digest or absorb. Fiber moderates the way your body digests and helps you control your blood sugar (blood sugar / glucose levels). Foods rich in fiber are vegetables, fruits, nuts of various kinds, legumes (beans, peas and lentils), flour obtained from whole wheat and wheat bran.

Foods that contain unsaturated fats

Foods that contain "good" fats are essential in a diet for diabetes. For example, foods that contain monounsaturated fats and polyunsaturated fats help keep your blood cholesterol under control. These foods can be avocados, almonds, pecans, regular nuts, olives and various healthy oils, such as olive oil, peanut oil and rapeseed oil. You should not overdo these fats, as all fats are high in calories.

Low protein foods

When it comes to treating diabetes, you need to start with a diet. There are certain foods that can help you balance the amount of glucose in your blood (blood sugar). Ideally, your meals should be rich in: protein, fiber and healthy fats. So foods that contain protein must exist in a balanced way in the diet for diabetes. Protein foods are salmon and poultry eggs, peas and figs. So, under the guidance of a nutritionist, you will know what kind of protein to include in your diet.

Foods high in fatty acids in the diet for diabetes

Fatty acids must also be found in the diet for diabetes. For example, the best advice is to eat fish meat at least twice a week. Fish can be a good alternative to those high-fat meats. For example, you can eat cod, tuna and halibut, which have less total fat, less saturated fat and less cholesterol than red and poultry. Fish such as salmon, mackerel, tuna and sardines are rich in Omega-3 fatty acids, which contribute to the health of your heart, reducing certain fats in the blood (such as triglycerides). Avoid fried fish and fish with a high level of mercury.

Foods to avoid in the diet for diabetes

Diabetes is a disease that increases your risk of suffering from heart disease (cardiovascular) and stroke, by accelerating the development of clogged arteries or arteries that are rigid, hardened by the deposition of atheroma plaques. That is why it is important to avoid certain foods, which can "work" in the opposite direction of your goal, to keep your heart healthy.

Processed foods

Processed foods have nothing to do with a diabetes diet either, especially since trans fats are a big enemy in this case. These types of fats are found in processed foods, in processed snacks, in cooked or baked foods, in various types of margarine and commercial fats. Avoid these products to maintain your health.

Foods high in cholesterol

Cholesterol is one of our enemies, not just an enemy of those with diabetes. That's why you need to keep in mind that foods high in cholesterol are not recommended in the diet for diabetes. Sources of cholesterol include high-fat dairy products and high-fat animal protein, egg yolks, liver and other animal organs. Try to set a goal or a goal and do not consume more than 200 mg of cholesterol per day.

Saturated fat foods

Saturated fats are not recommended in the diet for diabetes. High-fat dairy products and animal proteins such as beef, hot dogs, sausages and bacon contain saturated fats.

Foods with a high salt content

Sodium is an ingredient in sodium chloride, as is also known as table salt. When you suffer from diabetes, you must remember that foods with a high salt content should be avoided. So your goal or goal is to consume less than 2,300 mg of sodium per day, writes mayoclinic.org. However, if you also suffer from high blood pressure, you should try to consume less than 1,500 mg of sodium a day.

Foods that should be eaten in moderation for diabetes

The common name for food sugar is carbohydrates. Patients with diabetes are allowed to consume a certain amount of sugar per day and at each meal, depending on weight, physical activity, treatment and associated conditions.

Foods that may increase blood sugar and triglycerides, if consumed in excess, and the amount corresponding to a serving of 10 grams of sugar or 10 Carbohydrates:

1. Wholemeal bread, black, rye, graham, with bran, with seeds: 20 g = 1 slice

2. Whole grains, wheat flakes, oats, buckwheat, Psyllium, etc: 15 g = 1 tablespoon

3. Flour: Rice, Gray, Bulgur, Pasta, noodles, couscous: 50 g boiled = 1 tbsp

4. Legumes, Grains - Peas, Beans, Corn, Chickpeas, Lentils, Soybeans: 50 g cooked = 1 tbsp

5. Starch - White, red, sweet, purple potatoes: 50 g boiled = 1 tablespoon

6. Fruits with 20% sugar - Bananas, Grapes, Pears, Plums, Quince, Pomegranate, Mango: 50 g

7. Fruits with 10% sugar - Apples, Peaches, Nectarines, Cherries, Cherries, Apricots, Berries, Citrus - Pineapple, Oranges, Kiwi: 100 g

8. Fruit with 5% sugar - Watermelon, yellow, Grape-fruit, pomelo, sweetie, lemon: 150 g

9. Lactate Moi - Milk, yogurt, kefir, sana, Fresh cheese, pearls, cottage: 150g - 200 ml

Use the food scale and weigh all the food until you get used to the recommended portions and weights. To regulate your blood sugar, the most important thing is to have approximately the same amount of carbohydrates or carbohydrates at each meal, so that the antidiabetic, hypoglycemic treatment can be adjusted according to your choices and food preferences.

In general, a moderately hypoglycemic diet should contain about 160 grams of carbohydrates per day, divided into 3 main meals and 2 intermediate snacks.

Choose and combine foods as simply as possible

• 2 slices of bread (40 g) at each main meal

• 2 tablespoons potato / rice / pasta / polenta / berries (100 g in cooking) - for lunch

• 2 average fruits per day, between main meals, no later than 18.00

• 2 servings of dairy products / day (2 cups) per day, morning and evening, as needed

Fruits with a high fructose content

All fresh fruits are rich in vitamins and fiber, and this makes them a healthy part of any diet. However, some fruits contain more sugar than others. Bananas, melons and stone fruits such as peaches and nectarines are on the side with a high sugar content. These fruits can cause sudden increases in blood sugar more than any other, although this may not be the case for all patients. But you can replace fruits with a high fructose content with other fruits: Granny Smith apples, blueberries and other berries that have little fructose. It is important to eat fruit in moderation and not to combine it too often with peanut butter or cheese - even defatted. Test your blood sugar two hours after eating fruit to see how your body reacts.

Seeds

As you fill your plate at each meal, here's a little guide to keep in mind each time: half fill the plate with vegetables that don't contain much starch. Complete your meal with other healthy choices, such as whole grains, nuts and seeds, skim dairy products, lean protein and small portions of fresh fruit and healthy fat sources. But nutritionists tell us that seeds and nuts should be eaten in moderation.

Wholemeal pasta

Whole wheat pasta, considered a complex carbohydrate, is an excellent option for a diabetic, as long as it is eaten in moderation. You can look for pasta made from several cereals, which combines wheat with other types of cereals, but you should read the list of ingredients on the package to make sure they are made from whole wheat. Most pasta brands now offer you a wide range of products to choose from. The shape and size of the pasta makes them suitable for dishes such as soups, salads and side dishes.

Drinks in the diet for diabetes

Food is often in the spotlight when it comes to diabetes, but keep in mind that the drinks you drink can also affect your body weight and blood sugar. It is important to hydrate, and water is simply the best option you have when it comes to hydration.

Recommended drinks for diabetes

If you are tired of drinking only water, you can change your routine for diabetes by choosing unsweetened teas. Hot or cold, teas of all kinds ensure the diversity you need. Drink black tea, green tea or unsweetened herbal tea. You can drink mineral water or make infused water at home. To do this, you just need to put water in a container, in the refrigerator, with slices of cucumber, strawberries or fresh mint leaves, to get a soft drink with few calories. Simple coffee and tea contain very few calories and few carbohydrates and can be part of a healthy diet. That is why it is good not to add in coffee coffee, sugar, sweeteners and all kinds of toppings that have many calories and many carbohydrates, which have an impact on blood sugar (glucose).

The best options when it comes to recommended drinks for diabetes are:

• water or mineral water

• unsweetened tea (in which you can add a slice of lemon)

• light beer, small amounts of wine

• plain black coffee with skim milk or a sugar substitute.

Drinks forbidden to diabetics

Avoid or completely exclude sugary drinks, such as sour juices, fruit punch, energy drinks, sports drinks, sweet tea and other such drinks, with a high sugar content. These will increase your blood sugar and bring you a few hundred calories in one serving. Fruit juices are also not recommended in excess for diabetics, because they contain a lot of fructose.

The worst options (ie forbidden drinks) for diabetes are:

• sour drinks / juices

• regular beer, dessert wines, fruit drinks

• sweetened tea

• coffee with sugar and whipped cream

• different types of aromatic coffee and chocolate-based drinks

• energy drinks.

Drinks that should be consumed in moderation by people with diabetes or prone to diabetes. When choosing what to drink, there are a few things to consider that are relevant to your illness: diabetes. First of all, you need to think about whether your drink will affect your blood sugar and how much of that drink will affect your blood sugar. That is why it is good for certain drinks to be consumed in moderation and to take into account their caloric content.

• Milk - moderate carbohydrate content should be considered, especially in people with type 1 diabetes, if they drink close to or above 100 ml.

• Fruit juice - this is usually seen as a healthy option, but you should keep in mind that fruit juices or fresh fruits have a relatively high carbohydrate content. The calorie content of fruit juice is quite high, and therefore diabetics should consume it in moderation.

• Alcoholic beverages - when drinking alcohol, there are several factors to consider: how your drink will affect your blood sugar; how many calories does the drink contain; if alcohol interacts with any of the medicines you are taking. Alcohol can be responsible for raising and lowering blood sugar, so it is best to consume it in moderation or give it up altogether, especially since some medications interact with alcohol.

Recommended ways to prepare food for diabetes

In the diet for diabetes, there are some rules that you must follow when it comes to food preparation:

• Cook food with liquid fats instead of solids. Solid fats often include saturated fats, which you should limit, or trans fats, which you should avoid altogether. Many liquid fats, such as canola, corn, olives or grape seeds can be healthy when used in moderate amounts.

• Choose low-fat or low-fat dairy products. Many dairy products used in food preparation and baking are high in fat. You can reduce the fat content without compromising the taste of those dishes. Instead of whole milk, pour skim milk or milk with 1% fat. Instead of fermented sour cream, try plain skim yogurt, whipped milk or even low-fat cottage cheese.

• Generally use less fat. For many dishes, you can use 25% to 33% less fat than the amount specified in the recipe. Another trick: replace with apple puree or banana puree some or all of the fats in foods that require baking. Or if the recipe requires chocolate or chocolate flakes, try cocoa powder instead. When cooking a soup or stew, gather the fat that floats on the surface while it is still on the stove.

• Choose carbs wisely. Choose those carbohydrates that give you energy that lasts and that also gives you fiber. When a recipe tells you that you need white flour, white rice or other refined grains, try replacing the ingredients with whole wheat flour, brown rice or other whole grain products. You can use almond "flour", for example.

• Skip the sugar. This ingredient can quickly raise your blood sugar, unlike carbohydrates in vegetables or starchy products, which are absorbed much more slowly. Many times, you can reduce the amount of sugar or eliminate it completely without seriously affecting the taste or texture of a preparation, although you may need to add more flour. If you are using a sugar substitute, check the product label to make sure it is designed to be baked.

The role of regular meals for diabetics

Jumping over a table is not uncommon, but it is not a very wise thing, especially if you have diabetes. Maintaining your blood sugar at a normal level is vital to keeping the disease under control. What you eat - and what you don't eat - has a substantial effect on the amount of glucose that is present in the blood. Skipping meals puts you at high risk of developing hypoglycemia (low blood sugar), which can have dramatic repercussions. You need to eat regularly, at regular times, not to forget about snacks and to keep your blood sugar under control.

Having a balance between food intake and prescribed medications is vital if you are diabetic, whether we are talking about oral medications or insulin injections. Both methods of treatment require adherence to a strict and consistent schedule, ie to take your meals at regular times. You may not consume enough carbohydrates (which are broken down into glucose) if you skip meals. If you have missed one or more meals, especially if you are taking insulin injections or taking oral medications, this may increase your risk of developing very low blood sugar (hypoglycaemia), which can be dangerous for diabetics.

The role of proper hydration for diabetics

If you have diabetes you should drink as much water as possible. Water is an important part of any healthy diet. Drink enough water every day to prevent dehydration. If you have prediabetes, water is a healthy alternative to sugary juices, fruit juices and energy drinks. The amount of water you should drink each day depends on the size of your body, the level of physical activity and the climate in which you live. You can determine if you drink enough water by monitoring the volume of urine when you go to the bathroom. Also notice the color of the urine, as it should be pale yellow. People with diabetes have an increased risk of dehydration, because high blood glucose leads to decreased hydration in the body.

The symptoms of dehydration are:

• feeling thirsty

• headache

• dry mouth, dry eyes

• dizziness

• fatigue

• urine is dark yellow.

Diet plans for diabetes

If you suffer from this disease, it is important to put together all the information received from your specialist (in diabetes and metabolic diseases), as well as from the dietitian or nutritionist. First of all, you need to know that there are several different approaches to creating or building a diabetes diet from scratch, which are available to help you keep your blood sugar at normal. It is important to find a plan or a combination of the following methods for the diabetes diet to work for you.

Plate method 2-1-1

The method focuses on eating more vegetables. When preparing your plate, fill half of its surface with vegetables (which should not have a high starch content), such as spinach, carrots and tomatoes. Fill a quarter of a plate with a source of protein, such as tuna or lean pork. Fill the last quarter of the plate with a whole grain food (whole grains) or a starchy food. Add a portion of a fruit or a portion of dairy and a drink that can be unsweetened water or tea or unsweetened coffee.

Glycemic index measurement method

The glycemic index is a factor that you should not ignore if you have diabetes and if you have a special diet. Some people with diabetes use the method of measuring their glycemic index to choose the foods they eat, especially carbohydrates. This method classifies foods that contain carbohydrates, based on the effect that these foods have on the level of glucose in the blood (blood sugar).

Carbohydrate measurement method

You need to measure or count the carbohydrates in the foods you eat. Because carbohydrates break down into glucose, they have the greatest impact on your blood sugar (the amount of glucose in your blood). To help keep your blood sugar under control, eat about the same amount of carbohydrates every day at regular intervals, especially if you are taking prescription diabetes or injecting insulin.

The method of food lists for creating a daily diet

This method of food lists helps you a lot in creating a daily diet if you suffer from diabetes. It is recommended that you use the food list method (or food exchange system) to help you plan your main meals of the day and snacks in advance. The lists are organized into categories, such as: carbohydrates, protein sources and fats. A portion in a category is called a "choice." A food choice has almost the same amount of carbohydrates, protein, fat and calories - and the same effect on your blood sugar - as it has a portion of every other food in the same category. Thus, you could choose to eat half of a large corn or 65 g of cooked pasta for a choice from the category of starchy foods.

16 foods that help keep diabetes under control

Diabetes is a disease that doctors have placed in clear categories, depending on the cause of the disease, the factors that favor it, the way it is triggered and the way it affects our lives. People with diabetes are now much more likely to keep your disease under control than in previous years, when diabetes was not so well known and not as effectively treated.

1. Fatty fish such as salmon, sardines, herring, anchovies and mackerel, a source of Omega 3 fatty acids. Omega 3 acids are essential for heart health, lowering inflammation and regulating blood sugar.

2. Greens such as spinach, kale, lettuce and so on. They are a source of vitamin C, essential for people with diabetes. Vitamin C is antioxidant with anti-inflammatory power and with the effect of restoring damaged cells in the body.

3. Avocado is also on the list because it is high in fiber, low in calories and sugars. There are studies that show that avocado could even be involved in the prevention of diabetes because it would reduce insulin resistance, a problem that afflicts people with diabetes.

4. Eggs are also recommended for diabetics because they keep you hungry for a long time and then you don't go to foods that contain carbohydrates. Moreover, eggs increase good cholesterol, decrease inflammation, improve insulin sensitivity and support a low-carb diet, ideal for diabetics.

5. Chia seeds. They are ideal for people with diabetes because they are rich in fiber and they are perfect for diets and diabetes. Chia seeds lower blood sugar and keep you hungry for a long time. Moreover, chia seeds decrease inflammation in the body.

6. Legumes are also recommended in diabetes because they provide essential nutrients, vitamins and minerals, have a low glycemic index and can prevent diabetes.

There is a study done on more than 3,000 participants at high risk of cardiovascular disease in which those who consumed higher amounts of legumes were 35% less likely to develop diabetes.

7. Yogurt. Weak dairy products help reduce insulin resistance. Moreover, yogurt keeps you hungry for a long time due to the proteins it contains. This means that you can make sure you stay away from other foods for a long time.

8. Walnuts are also super ideal for diabetics and more. Walnuts have very small amounts of carbohydrates, which is especially important for people with diabetes. Walnuts lower inflammation in the body, lower bad cholesterol, raise good cholesterol, prevent obesity and maintain optimal blood sugar levels.

9. Broccoli is also recommended in diabetes because it has few carbohydrates and enough fiber to keep us hungry. Moreover, broccoli contains antioxidants that fight free radicals and help repair damaged cells in the body. Broccoli contains nutrients that prevent inflammation in the body, reduce insulin resistance and maintain optimal blood glucose levels due to sulforaphane, the same compound tested and retested to confirm the potential to fight cancer.

10. Extra virgin olive oil is essential in any diet and especially for people suffering from diabetes because this food lowers bad cholesterol, increases good cholesterol (which lowers bad cholesterol, as in a wonderful cycle), lowers triglyceride levels, inflammation and prevents obesity. Moreover, olive oil contains antioxidants that fight cell damage.

11. Flax seeds. We normally eat them because they have fiber, which is exactly what we need if we suffer from diabetes. Fiber provides satiety, rich bacterial flora in the gut, Omega 3 fatty acids that fight inflammation and obesity, heart disease and more.

12. Apple cider vinegar. There are studies that show that apple cider vinegar could improve blood sugar levels. Use diluted, in plain water, one tablespoon of apple cider vinegar in a glass of water, maximum 2 tablespoons a day, added gradually, not at first.

13. Strawberries are ideal for people suffering from diabetes due to anthocyanins, compounds that reduce inflammation in the body, prevent obesity and heart disease, regulate blood sugar levels. Moreover, strawberry polyphenols can improve insulin sensitivity, which is especially important for diabetics. In time, insulin resistance may occur, meaning that the cells are no longer receptive to insulin and then can no longer receive the sugar that is in the blood. Sugar must reach the cells and be used to release energy. If the insulin fails to send the sugar to the cells, it remains in the blood.

14. Garlic lowers blood sugar and cholesterol. It is said that we should eat at least a clove of garlic every day, in whatever form we want. Even garlic is a natural remedy that my grandmothers used for absolutely any disease in the world.

15. Pumpkin and squash. They are low in carbohydrates, rich in fiber, have low glycemic index and compounds that can control obesity and cholesterol. There are studies that say that pumpkins and squash can improve blood sugar levels in the body.

16. Shirataki noodles, rich in fiber extracted from konjac root, are foods that maintain optimal blood sugar levels, keep you hungry for long periods of time and have a low glycemic index.

5

CELEBRITY DIETS

1. From the secrets of Victoria Beckham

It is always supple, full of energy and has a radiant skin. And this even if he went through four pregnancies and is not long in his early youth. Victoria Beckham is another clear example that nothing comes naturally. When it comes to a healthy lifestyle, the star is one of the most disciplined celebrities. "I have high expectations of my body. And I'm never sick. You have to be good with your body, if you have expectations from it ", Victoria explained at one point about her lifestyle. Therefore, she regularly exercises and is very careful about what she drinks and eats. Beyond the usual set of rules, which she strictly follows, she has a few more tricks that help her stay in such great shape.

Consume apple cider vinegar in the morning

The star revealed that she takes two tablespoons of apple cider vinegar every morning as soon as she wakes up. Distributing a picture of the bottle of vinegar on her Instagram account, she encouraged fans to "be brave", confessing that she starts every day with its administration, on an empty stomach. Her ritual does not end here, the dose of vinegar is followed by freshly squeezed lemon in boiling water.

She makes green smoothies

The drink she loves to make is known in the Beckham family home as the "green monster" for breakfast. To make this smoothie, Victoria uses a nutritious mixture of apples, kiwi, lemon, spinach, broccoli and chia seeds.

She eats a lot of avocados

Victoria Beckham said she is a big avocado consumer. Not only does it include it in the menu every day, but it also gives it a special privilege in terms of quantity. Eat three or four avocados a day. He said that he does this little abuse to keep his skin healthy. Admittedly, the effect is obvious. Victoria has an impeccable complexion and is often assailed with questions about how she takes care of him.

Victoria Beckham relies on the so-called "5 hands" diet. It is eaten 5 times a day, preferably at the same hours. The amount of food consumed should not exceed a handful. It is preferable to eat low-calorie foods with a low glycemic index. Maximum calories that can be consumed in a day is 1200 (1500 calories for men).

FIVE diet: nutritional principles

This diet can be followed for weeks on end, as it does not pose any health risks. But it involves a great diversification of food, so it is possible that at first you will find it harder to adjust, being necessary to learn where to buy certain products, to replenish your stocks of healthy food, to discover how to store them, how to prepare them, etc. The FIVE diet recommends drinking only water, in which you can add lemon juice, fruit slices or a knife tip of baking soda.

The menu of the FIVE diet

FIVE diet: breakfast

At breakfast you can consume the only cup of coffee allowed per day. You can sweeten it, add milk (but NOT condensed) and drink it only after meals.

Foods allowed for breakfast, only in the suggested combinations (choose only one option):

- Fresh vegetable salad with seeds (without oil, dressing or any other addition except salt and pepper). You can season with vegetables (parsley, dill, basil, thyme, mint, etc.).

- Cheese salad with fruits, nuts and arugula;

- A simple yogurt;

- Grilled chicken breast with fresh vegetables.

FIVE diet: the first snack of the day

This snack takes place around 10-11, being represented by a small meal between breakfast and lunch. You can consume, to choose between:

- A banana;

- A yogurt

- An apple or other fruit, provided you have lunch in at least an hour (otherwise you get bloated)

Diet FIVE: lunch

You can consume, at your choice:

- A bowl of soup or broth, no oil in the recipe and no bread;

- Grill with grilled or steamed vegetables;

- Large vegetable salad with cheese or tuna;

- Omelette made in water with fresh vegetables;

At this meal you will not eat bread and you will NOT put oil in salads.

FIVE diet: afternoon snack

You can consume a variant of the following:

- A cup of tea;

- A cup of warm milk with honey;

- Fresh fruits or vegetables as such or in salads;

- Unripe seeds and nuts (like radishes);

- Candied fruit (not more than one cup)

FIVE diet: dinner

At dinner you can consume, at your choice, the same options you have at lunch.

The diet minimizes fats in the diet, but also starches and sugars. So the fats are provided by the meat grill, oilseeds and seeds, avoiding oils, butter, sour cream, etc. Carbohydrates are provided to the body from fruits and vegetables, but also honey.

Thus, the FIVE diet involves the consumption of healthy fats and good quality carbohydrates, having obvious effects on the figure, but also on health.

2. Kim Kardashian

After the birth of her daughter North, Kim Kardashian turned to the Atkins diet, low in carbohydrates, which promotes the consumption of good fats: any type of meat, fish and seafood, eggs, cabbage, spinach, broccoli, asparagus, butter, cheese, cream, yogurt, milk, almonds, macadamia nuts, walnuts, sunflower seeds, extra virgin olive oil, coconut oil, avocado and avocado oil.

The Atkins diet is considered one of the most effective diets and is based on a low carb diet. A daily menu for a person on an Atkins diet is based on healthy proteins, vegetables and fats. The good part is that you can lose weight without counting calories, as long as the portions are a reasonable size. The Atkins diet has four important phases, the first (induction) being the hardest: it is the stage in which you are allowed to consume only 20 grams of carbohydrates per day.

Atkins Diet Phase 1: Induction

It is the strictest phase of the Atkins diet, in which you are allowed to eat only 20 grams of carbohydrates per day. If you want to keep the diet "as per the book", in the induction phase you should avoid fruits, bread, cereals, vegetables with high starch content, dairy products (except cheese and butter), alcohol. Your diet at this stage should be based on protein and green leafy vegetables.

Atkins Diet Phase 2: Continue to lose weight

At this stage, you can gradually introduce foods with higher carbohydrate content, such as berries, legumes, oilseeds, tomato juice, yogurt. You can eat between 25 and 50 grams of carbohydrates a day. The second phase must be kept until you manage to lose 4 kilograms since you started the diet.

Atkins Diet Phase 3: Pre-Maintenance

At this stage, gradually reintroduce other carbohydrates into your diet: fruits, starchy vegetables, whole grains. Now you can eat between 50 and 80 grams of carbohydrates a day. Phase three lasts at least a month from the moment you reach the desired weight.

Atkins Diet Phase 4: Maintaining

Once you reach the ideal weight, continue with a diet in which carbohydrates do not have a significant percentage: 80-100 grams per day.

Atkins diet: daily menu

What foods should you avoid if you are on the Atkins diet:

Foods that contain sugar

Cereals

Vegetable oils

Trans fats

"Dietary" foods

Vegetables and fruits with high carbohydrate content (in induction)

Vegetables and fruits with high starch content (in induction)

Legumes (induction)

What foods are recommended in the Atkins diet:

Meat: beef, pork, lamb, chicken, bacon, etc.

Fatty fish and seafood: salmon, trout, sardines, etc.

Eggs

Vegetables with low carbohydrate content: kale, spinach, broccoli, asparagus, etc.

Non-fat dairy products: butter, cheese, sour cream, yogurt

Nuts and seeds

Healthy fats (extra virgin olive oil, coconut oil, avocado and avocado oil)

Atkins diet: daily menu

MONTHS

Breakfast: Vegetable omelette, prepared with butter or coconut oil

Lunch: Grilled fish (mackerel, salmon, herring, sardines) with vegetables / tuna salad

Dinner: Hamburger without bun, served with vegetables and salsa / ketchup sauce

TUESDAY

Breakfast: Bacon and eggs.

Lunch: Hamburger left over from the previous evening or pork steak with vegetables

Dinner: salmon made in butter, with vegetables.

WEDNESDAY

Breakfast: Boiled eggs with vegetables

Lunch: Shrimp salad with a little olive oil or salad with feta cheese

Dinner: Grilled chicken with vegetables

THURSDAY:

Breakfast: Cheese with vegetables

Lunch: A low carb sausage with salad

Dinner: Steak and vegetables

FRIDAY:

Breakfast: Smoked salmon with vegetables

Lunch: Chicken salad with a little olive oil

Dinner: Pork chop with vegetables

SATURDAY:

Breakfast: Cremvust low carb with vegetables and / or tuna salad

Lunch: Baked pudding with cauliflower, butter, eggs and grated cheese

Dinner: Baked meatballs with vegetables

SUNDAY:

Breakfast: Omelette with mushrooms

Lunch: Salad with bacon, spinach, cheese with mold (30g), cherry tomatoes and broccoli or grilled mackerel with broccoli

Dinner: Grilled chicken wings with spinach

3. Christina Aguilera

The singer says she has an unusual diet: she eats something crispy, soft, hot and cold every day. Also, the food should be the same color - if you choose white on Monday, then you will eat cabbage, white phallus and cow's cheese. Although it sounds strange, it is difficult to doubt the effectiveness of such a diet when we look at its perfect figure.

4. Madonna

Madonna looks great for her age. That's because while others eliminate calories, she completely excludes them. Madonna's diet is based on the assumption that air is enough to support the body's activity. The diva cooks, but does not enjoy the dishes, but only smells the food and consumes only salt water soup. He certainly does not practice this method all the time, but he uses it when necessary.

5. Nicole Kidman

After giving birth, Nicole Kidman had to follow a rather harsh diet for her future film projects. The diet consisted of one boiled egg for breakfast, one for lunch and two for dinner. With this diet, the actress managed to lose more weight than expected. Verdict: It works, but you can't resist such a diet for long.

6. Heidi Klum

Heidi Klum preferred the diet in which she ate every 3 hours, the last meal being at 7 p.m. Under this diet, the model drinks a protein-rich shake for breakfast, followed three hours away by an omelet prepared from four egg whites plus vegetables. The third meal of the day consisted of steamed broccoli and grilled skinless chicken breast, after three hours 8 almonds, and in the evening a turkey steak with chilli or another protein shake.

7. Cameron Diaz

Cameron Diaz avoids all white carbohydrates, such as rice, pasta, bread or biscuits. Her method is very healthy and effective in the weight loss process because all these foods contain a lot of sugar, and consumed, it would mean that the body would first process this sugar, instead of fat. If these carbohydrates are removed from the diet, however, the body goes directly to burning fat. At the same time, Cameron Diaz avoids sweet drinks, which makes the diet even more efficient. And to return to carbohydrates, the actress admits that she still has a diet rich in carbohydrates, because she eats a lot of fruits and vegetables.

8. Jennifer Aniston

It is not known exactly what is the secret behind Jennifer Aniston's diet, but for 10 years, the actress ate the same salad, every day, at lunch, a Cobb salad. A very healthy choice, Cobb salad often contains lettuce leaves, tomato slices, a boiled egg, pieces of grilled meat and diced cheese, plus avocado. More precisely, such a salad ensures the optimal need for good quality fiber and carbohydrates, low protein, but also vitamins and minerals. No wonder, then, why all these years, Jennifer Aniston has not struggled with too many weight fluctuations.

9. Jennifer Lopez

One of Jennifer Lopez's diet secrets is the habit of eating in the morning. It may seem trivial, but breakfast plays an important role in most diets, so this habit, responsible for putting your metabolism into action, should be respected by everyone. The artist says she eats in the morning in the first 30 minutes after waking up, and the meal is usually composed of oatmeal with a little milk and fresh fruit or egg white omelet, which is very rich in protein and full.

10. Katy Perry

Katy Perry says her diet secret is that she eats little and often. In addition to the main meals, the singer eats up to three snacks a day, but they do not exceed 100 calories each. Katy believes that this keeps her metabolism running throughout the day and admits that it is much easier for her to eat healthy this way. Her favorite snacks include vegetable slices, strawberries, or whole grain biscuits.

11. Kelly Osbourne

Kelly Osbourne has lost a lot of weight lately, and the recipe for her success was based on a lot of sports and a balanced diet. However, one of his tricks was to eat half an apple in the evening, before bed, so that his metabolism would continue to burn calories. Thus, the singer says that, although she violated the rules of not eating before bed, in her case she feels that this trick really worked.

12. Kristen Stewart

Kristen Stewart said her diet tricks include low-calorie snacks, such as whole-grain biscuits or nuts and seeds, high-fiber, high-carb, high-protein breakfast, such as a low-fat ham sandwich. turkey and salad or an omelette made from egg whites and fresh vegetables, but also meals based only on raw foods, often fresh salads, garnished with all kinds of vegetables.

6

TIPS AND RECOMMENDATIONS

The best tips and secrets that work in weight loss diets are: watch the meal schedule, avoid eating chaotically, even if you take a simple snack with an apple or a few nuts. As soon as you start a diet, you must have a rigorous schedule and follow it. Respect the number of servings and calories Regardless of the diet, be sure to eat only as much as is allowed, because the foods are combined in such a way as to help you cope with the early stages, when you often feel hungry.

Do not eat in the evening, if you have breakfast at 9 o'clock, your last meal / snack must be at 5 o'clock, ie eight hours after the first meal of the day. Do not exceed the interval of eight hours and do not eat in the evening after 17 or 18 hours, it is the golden rule in any diet to lose weight. Be careful how you combine food. Prepare meals as simple as possible, with one or two dietary preparations, according to the menu of your diet. Do not combine too many ingredients and foods, even if they are on the allowed list. If you also eat soup, steak, salad, toast and a fruit dessert you will not lose weight too soon, even if they are prepared dietary. Choose only two dishes for lunch and one for dinner. Don't climb the scales every day. If you have started a diet, you do not have to weigh yourself daily.

The results may be delayed and you will be disappointed, and the temptation to give up will be great. Weigh yourself once every three days or only once a week, especially if you are on a long-term diet. Set a clear goal to lose x pounds in 3 days or 7 days and be persevering. When the scale shows that you have reached your goal, you will be more optimistic and determined to continue your diet. Drink plenty of plain water no matter what weight loss diets you follow. As healthy and delicious as they may seem, fresh fruit juices or teas may contain sugars or glucose that delay the effects of diets.

The best advice is to drink plenty of plain water every day, as much as your body needs and an extra glass. Find a pleasant sports activity, you need exercise, especially if you are sedentary and can not lose weight too fast. Choose a light sport, gymnastics, long walks, bike rides, dancing, but whatever you choose, make a program to exercise every day for at least 30 minutes. No diet works wonders if you do not tone your muscles and skin through daily exercise. Calories and weight loss diets, always pay attention to calorie intake in weight loss diets.

The diet you want to follow should not contain absurd rules and starve you until you fall off your feet. It should be a balanced diet and suitable for your metabolism, but any diet requires strict calorie control. Regardless of the diet you choose, you definitely need to greatly reduce bread, pastries, cakes, fried and fatty foods, alcohol or fatty cheeses. To lose weight, at the end of each day you need to burn more calories than you consume. The bigger the difference, the faster you lose weight, but to a point where the metabolism can be unbalanced.

In general, women should have a consumption of 1200 calories per day, and men, 1800 calories. Ideally, you should reduce your usual number of calories by 500 daily and you will lose half a kilogram in a week. A daily decrease in the number of calories by 1000 can lead to a weight loss of one kilogram per week. When you lose weight gradually and calculated, your metabolism helps you and the risk of losing weight again is much lower.

Tip 1: Don't give up diet because of hunger

Whatever diet you follow, do not give up because, over time, you feel that you are too hungry.

"Hunger is one of the reasons many people fail to follow a weight loss plan for more than a few weeks. Don't be fooled by hunger and remember that when you eat less fat cells release more hunger hormones." "The best diets that help you control your hunger and appetite are those based on high protein and low carbohydrate intake," said Dawn Noe, a dietitian at Cleveland Clinical Wellness Institute. Avoid eating white bread, pretzels, muffins or donuts for breakfast because they are rich in processed carbohydrates. Instead, opt for high-protein foods, such as eggs or yogurt mixed with chia seeds and berries. You will find that the feeling of satiety lasts for a long time.

Tip 2: Eat high-fiber carbohydrates

Fiber-rich carbohydrates are the so-called good carbohydrates that do not make you fat. Fiber improves blood sugar control, helps lower cholesterol and reduces the risk of chronic diseases such as diabetes, colorectal cancer and heart disease.

High fiber foods:

• Vegetables and legumes: broccoli, spinach, Brussels sprouts, sweet potatoes, dried beans, lentils

• Fruits: apples, pears, berries, oranges

American dietitians encourage the consumption of fiber and recommend avoiding, as much as possible, bad carbohydrates, such as: white bread, pasta, pretzels, pastries, candy, carbonated juices.

Tip 3: Focus on adopting healthy behaviors

It is very easy to get discouraged and give up the diet when you focus only on the number of kilograms. Experts recommend, instead, that you focus on making more healthy food choices, keeping your portion size under control, and exercising moderately every day. Once you adopt these behaviors, you will begin to lose weight. Instead of trying to lose a pound a week, set goals such as eating a serving (cup) of vegetables for dinner or walking for 20 minutes each day. It is also important to keep a food diary to monitor changes in lifestyle, diet, exercise and weight. This way, at the end of each week, you will know if you need to work harder to achieve your goals.

Tip 4: Make sure your diet is based on vegetables and fruits

Each person, depending on their needs and preferences, opts for a certain weight loss plan. Numerous diets and diets are available, but each of them must be based mainly on vegetables. Eat starchy vegetables with confidence: broccoli, cauliflower, kale, cucumber and Chinese cabbage. It also includes berries, apples and pears in the diet. A diet based on vegetables and fruits not only helps in weight loss, but also prevents the onset of chronic diseases, such as diabetes, cardiovascular disease, etc. Vegetables and fruits contain a variety of vitamins, minerals and phytonutrients, including fiber and water, increasing the feeling of satiety.

Tip 5: No food is 100% forbidden

When you divide food into "good" and "bad", you automatically focus on foods that you should not eat, but that you crave. Usually, the more a food is "forbidden", the more you think about it. The advice of American experts is to try to focus on eating healthy foods in the proportion of 80% -90%. This habit, combined with a constant exercise program, will lead in the long run to weight loss. In addition, in this way, you give yourself more freedom to occasionally enjoy high-calorie foods without feeling guilty. The feeling of guilt generated by eating "forbidden" foods acts like a snowball in the formation of unhealthy emotions in childhood, adolescence and even adulthood.

Tip 6: Consume calories wisely

If your diet consists mainly of foods rich in sugar, salt, saturated fats and trans fats, which can be addictive, you can develop serious cravings for low-calorie foods with low nutritional value. Over time, this eating behavior leads to weight gain or difficulties in reducing the number of kilograms. Eat foods rich in low protein, healthy fats and fiber: eggs, skinless chicken breast or turkey, beans, lentils, skim milk, tuna, salmon, tofu and other soy foods, nuts, peanuts, almonds, cashews . You will feel satisfied throughout the day and you will have less "cravings". In addition, you will consume fewer calories, which will lead to weight loss.

Tip 7: Plan today what you will eat tomorrow

Planning meals in advance helps you resist the urge to eat the first foods you see in front of your eyes when you are hungry, including in the evening before dinner. Once you feel hungry, you run the risk of eating high-calorie foods with fewer nutrients. Determine what you will eat the next evening. In this way, you have enough time to thaw food and, the next day, you will prepare food much faster, without having to quench your hunger with unhealthy foods.

7

A TRUE STORY ABOUT THE HARSH REALITY OF EXTRA POUNDS

The extra pounds are a big burden, a weight that you have to carry with you every day wherever you go. I remember how hard it was for me in the summer to carry those pounds through the heat that melted me, but it was just as hard for me in the winter when the weight was even heavier because the pounds were covered by other pounds of clothes.

I never took any diet seriously, they were all too heavy and involved a lot of physical effort but also starvation. I was pleased with my situation. When I managed to make a boyfriend who wasn't so unhappy with how I looked, I started to be even more careless. We both ate in the evening, in front of the TV, no matter how we looked, and he was as fat as I was.

I felt good about doing all my food cravings at any time and I didn't realize I was doing myself a lot of harm. Only a miracle could have given me a boost and done something for me, for my health and the way I look. And this miracle happened, but it came with moments of horror.

I was at work, I am an accountant at a company, when a colleague called and announced that he could not come to work because he felt very ill. A few hours later, my colleague announced that he was in the hospital, he was infected with the dreaded covid virus and we all had to go for tests because we came in contact with him. Suddenly I seemed to realize that I did not feel the taste of coffee, I who am a great lover of coffee. When I got to the hospital, my suspicion was confirmed, and I was infected with this virus. Several colleagues were confirmed positively. We did not have any serious symptoms, so we all went home and took the appropriate treatment and were isolated.

When I got home, I started to feel worse, so my boyfriend got really scared and called for help. I didn't know about myself for a few days, I just remember that I couldn't breathe or go back to bed from side to side, I needed the help of two nurses.

When I started to recover, the nurses told me every day that I was very lucky to escape because obese people lost the fight against the virus. It was the first time I promised myself that I would do something for myself, to take care of my health and my body.

I recovered from this difficult period, but I was left with some psychological sequelae. I never let a day go by that I didn't do something for myself. I set out to climb the scales every Sunday and weigh 3 kg each time. I bought a short, gorgeous dress, size 38 and said that until I put on this dress I will not stop. I cleaned the fridge, threw away everything that was unhealthy. I stocked up on a lot of fruits, vegetables, fish, rice, diet yogurts and lean meat. I made a schedule to eat three meals a day, both, the last being at a maximum of 6 pm. I definitely gave up sweets and bread. I focused a lot on vegetables and fruits. At lunch we ate a piece of boiled meat with lots of vegetables and salad. I also involved my boyfriend in this program, we supported each other. In the evening we took an hour's walk, we walked for an hour without stopping.

The determination and the will were so strong that I never felt that I could not continue and I will give in to food cravings. There were many improvements in my daily life, I looked better and better, I was losing weight and I seemed to be rejuvenating. I still haven't been able to put on that dress, but I knew that day would come too. The relationship with my boyfriend became full of passion, I had romantic evenings where I made love and I felt so wanted. One day my boyfriend confessed to me that I was the most beautiful woman and he never thought I would look so good.

This wonderful period of my life reached its peak when my boyfriend proposed to me to go to the sea for a few days. I gladly accepted and enjoyed my new figure in a swimsuit. One evening, while we were walking on the beach, my boyfriend told me to close my eyes a little, I listened to him, and when I opened them he was in front of me on his knees and holding a beautiful ring in his hand, he asked me if I wanted to be his wife, I said yes with all my heart.

The civil wedding took place after a few months, during which time I managed to lose weight so I wore that red dress. Nothing is accidental, everything happens for a purpose.

An unfortunate event was the impetus that led me to take a stand on how I look. I was lucky to have a good time, but there were also many cases when young people lost their lives due to extra pounds. It is very important to have a balance in everything you do, nothing should exceed a limit.

The fight with extra pounds is very hard, but the will and ambition must be the ones that overcome and overcome any obstacle. It's so beautiful when you see that you manage to win a fight. Fight for yourself, for the way you look and think that you have to eat to live, you do not live to eat and to guide you in life after satisfying your appetites.

You eat little and love a lot.